Gluten-Free Kids:

A Quick Start Guide for a Healthy Kids Diet

by Jennifer Wells

Table of Contents

Introduction 1

CHAPTER 1: What Is Gluten? 4

CHAPTER 2: What Exactly Are Celiac Disease and Gluten Intolerance and What Are Their Symptoms?.........................8

CHAPTER 3: Is Gluten Bad for My Child…and Me?...........13

CHAPTER 4: How Does a Gluten-Free Diet Compare to a Grain-Free Diet?...20

CHAPTER 5: Where Do I Begin?...24

CHAPTER 6: What Will My Pantry and Refrigerator Look Like without Gluten?..34

CHAPTER 7: What Does a Gluten-Free Shopping List Look Like? 36

CHAPTER 8: How Do I Talk to My Child about Gluten Sensitivity? 48

CHAPTER 9: What Do Meals and Snacks Look Like for My Child? 52

CHAPTER 10: How Do I Deal with School Lunches? 56

CHAPTER 11: How Do We Eat Out Safely?.........................60

CHAPTER 12: Is There a Link between Gluten, ADHD and Other Neurological Problems?..64

In Closing..69

Additional Resources 72

Acknowledgements 73

About the Author 74

Endnotes 76

Resources

Additional works by Jennifer Wells.

Going Gluten Free:
A Quick Start Guide for a Gluten-Free Diet

Juice for Health:
The Benefits of Juicing for Health and Wellness

Top 10 Tips to Help You Lose Weight

Introduction

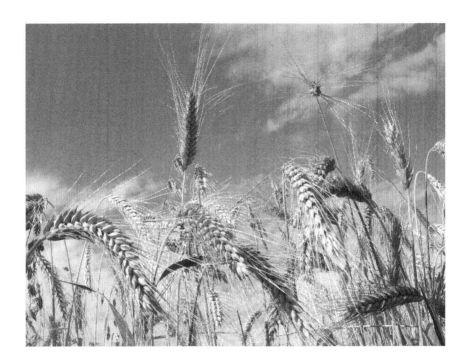

Children are incredibly fond of eating foods that are sweet, fatty and high in carbohydrates. Notice how they seem to gravitate toward candies, chocolates, cakes, ice cream, chips, spaghetti, and macaroni and cheese. Though many children appear to handle these foods without negative consequences, other children do not.

In a growing body of research, gluten sensitivity and its effects in children are on the rise. According to author Michelle Matte in her article entitled, "Gluten Sensitivity in Children," gluten has been found to trigger neurological disorders like attention deficit hyperactive disorder, as well as being linked to various learning disorders and even developmental delays.[1]

If these results were not bothersome enough, she also points out that gluten sensitivity has been linked to respiratory disorders, lack of nutrition, constipation, skin irritations, and depression.[2]

While it appears that many children outgrow their sensitivity to gluten around the age of five,[3] researchers and parents alike are beginning to look at gluten sensitivity as one of the possible explanations for the rise of allergies in children.

If you are a parent with a child that suffers from some of the medical conditions I have just mentioned, you will be interested in the information presented here. When a child is found to be sensitive to gluten, the treatment is a gluten-free diet. This can prove difficult because there are so many foods in our diets that contain gluten.

You will discover gluten in many cereals, pastas, and breads; however, it can also "hide" in foods like marinades, potato chips, and candies. Fortunately, more and more products are being produced that are gluten-free as an effort to help meet the demand of parents concerned about the health of their children.

Come along with me and discover:

— What gluten is

— What symptoms to look for if you suspect your child is sensitive to gluten

— Find out how to recognize gluten in food products

— Discover strange places where gluten can "hide"

— Connect with helpful organizations that will support and guide you as you learn more about celiac disease and gluten allergies

While the information presented here is certainly not an exhaustive resource, it will give you important facts about gluten and an organized way of creating a gluten-free diet for your kids. It will guide you so you will know which areas to tackle first, how to clean out your pantry and refrigerator, help you with snack and lunch ideas for your kids, and teach you what items you can put on—and take off—your shopping list.

If you suspect your child is sensitive to gluten or they have been diagnosed with gluten intolerance or celiac disease, then this information will help you tremendously as you begin to create a gluten-free diet that will nurture and restore the health of your child.

In the next section, I am going to tell you exactly what gluten is and the grains that contain it.

CHAPTER 1:
What Is Gluten?

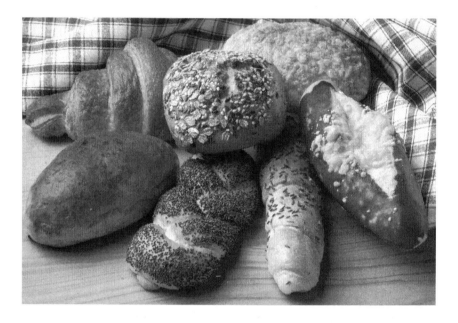

I believe it is important for you to know what gluten is and how it affects your child's body. Let me first define it and then share with you the grains that contain it.

Grains are classified as carbohydrates and about 10 to 15 percent of a kernel of grain is comprised of protein. Often referred to as the "germ" of the wheat, it is this part of the grain that will become a new plant. While varying from plant to plant, the most plentiful protein found in grains is gluten. In wheat specifically, gluten makes up about 80% of the protein.

When water is added to flour that is made from ground-up wheat kernels, the gluten becomes an elastic, sticky, and gooey substance. Then when kneading occurs during bread making, kneading causes the gluten to form long and flexible strands throughout the dough. Once the yeast is added to the dough, these gluten strands capture the gases released by the yeast and the dough rises. Subsequently, as the dough cooks in the oven, the heat from the baking process causes the strands of the gluten protein to harden in place and allows the dough to remain in a solid, heightened form. These properties of gluten are what give bread its strength and texture.

Gluten is responsible for the chewiness you enjoy in different types of breads. For instance, think of French bread with its hard outer crust and chewy texture inside. Gluten makes this possible. Now imagine the softness and light airy texture of a birthday cake. It is nothing like French bread because their differences are determined by how much the gluten is developed before it is cooked.

To create the chewiness found in French bread, the gluten is kneaded extensively; however, for a birthday cake, you want very little of the gluten to be developed. Additionally, without gluten, foods like bagels, pizza, doughnuts and yeast breads would not exist as we know them today.

When you are trying to determine which flours contain gluten, the list consists mainly the following grains:

— Spelt

— Kamut

— Wheat

— Rye

— Graham

— Semolina

— Triticale

— Einkorn

— Durum

— Barley

— Farro, and

— Bulgur

While oats do not contain gluten naturally, they do contain avenin. According to Dr. Rodney Ford, physician and pediatric allergy specialist, avenin is a protein that is similar in its properties to gluten, but fortunately, rarely causes a person to exhibit any adverse reactions to this type of protein.[4]

However, you will still need to be careful when buying products made with oats because oats are often processed commercially and can easily become contaminated with gluten because of its exposure to other grains containing gluten. Great care must be taken to keep grains separated during processing and storing. This must occur in order to eliminate cross-contamination of gluten grains with non-gluten grains such as oats.

Now that we have talked about what gluten is and its prevalence in various grains, it is time to talk about what gluten intolerance is and what its symptoms look like.

CHAPTER 2:
What Exactly Are Celiac Disease and Gluten Intolerance and What Are Their Symptoms?

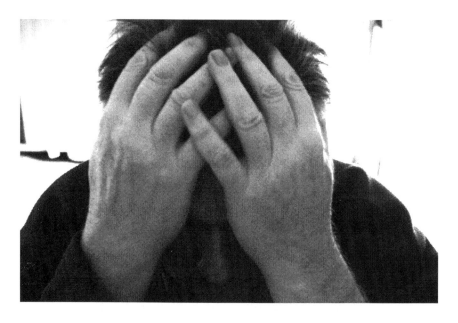

Let us say that you have reason to suspect that something is not right with your child's health. You notice a change in their behavior; they complain about headaches; their stomach hurts oftentimes after they eat.

To begin to sort out what might be happening, let us first discuss what celiac disease is and how it can affect your child's body.

While celiac disease was first described nearly two thousand years ago,[5] it has only been within the past few decades that the link between gluten and this chronic, debilitating disease has become clear. According to the Gluten Free Network, approximately 15% of the US population has some form of celiac disease or gluten intolerance,[6] making it clear that this health issue clearly affects a large number of people!

Celiac disease is an autoimmune condition. It is where your child's own immune system attacks normal cells within their body. These antibodies attack the lining of your child's small intestine and damage the small finger-like projections called "villi." With repeated damage, these villi begin to weaken and their ability to absorb nutrients from your child's ingestion of food is lessened. This means that celiac disease is also a disease of mal-absorption that can eventually result in malnutrition.

Along with this mal-absorption, the lining of your child's small intestine also becomes "leaky." If your child has celiac disease, antibodies form against one of the proteins of gluten known as gliadin. When gliadin is eaten, it in turn activates a protein in your child's gut known as zonulin, resulting in gaps that form between the cells of the intestinal lining. Once these gaps are formed, a huge amount of stomach bacteria and improperly digested wheat proteins can enter into your child's bloodstream that normally wouldn'rt.[7] Consequently, it really does not matter what level of sensitivity your child may have, for when it is subjected to gliadin found in wheat, it can create havoc in your child's digestive and immune systems.

If your child has celiac disease – and to a lesser extent, gluten sensitivity – whenever he eats a product that has gluten in it, it triggers an autoimmune response. This attack can cause inflammation in many organ systems wherever the antibodies find similar proteins to attack. Because their body is literally fighting against itself, certain side effects will result, yet they may not even realize the results are due to their gluten intake.

At this point, it is important to note that whenever a child is diagnosed with celiac disease, it becomes necessary for the child to remain on a gluten-free diet for the rest of their life in order to avoid debilitating symptoms. Gluten sensitivity is a type of allergy your child will never outgrow as he might some other food allergies.[8]

If your child is gluten intolerant, it can be difficult to diagnose because the onset can be slower than it is with celiac disease and the causes and symptoms can cover a wide range. Additionally, the symptoms of gluten intolerance and gluten sensitivity are not as severe as celiac disease. The most common symptoms to look for in your child if you suspect gluten allergies are:

— Constipation

— Diarrhea

— Eczema and various skin rashes

— Nausea

— Vomiting

— Cramping

— Weight loss and even failure to thrive

— Stools that have a foul odor

— Fatigue

— Headaches

In addition to a wide range of symptoms, both gluten intolerance and celiac disease can worsen due to infections, stress, and surgery.

If you think your child may be experiencing symptoms of celiac disease and gluten intolerance:

— First, make a list of the symptoms your child is having as well as any negative behaviors you observe. Because there are so many possibilities involved in the symptoms experienced by children with this allergy or disease, it is best not to compare your child even with other children you know to have gluten issues.

— Secondly, keep a food journal of the foods your child eats. It would be a good idea to write down everything your child eats for a two-week period. This will be very helpful for a qualified physician as they work toward making a diagnosis. Be sure to note any problems with behavior or physical symptoms displayed after any particular foods are consumed. In addition, do not eliminate gluten from their diet leading up to an appointment with a physician because you do not want the possibility of this condition to go undetected.

— Finally, make an appointment with a qualified physician and share your concerns with him. During the consultation, request testing.

Taking some of these necessary steps will start a process of helping you and your child discover whether he may be sensitive to gluten or not.

Now that we have discussed symptoms of celiac disease and gluten allergies, let us move on to a discussion about why you want to eliminate gluten from your child's diet and the steps involved in this process.

CHAPTER 3:
Is Gluten Bad for My Child...and Me?

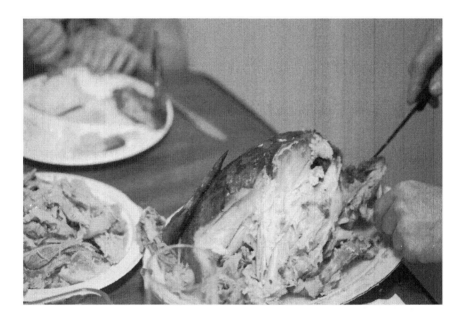

Eliminating gluten and grains from your child's diet may seem overwhelming at first. Discovering which grains are gluten-free and learning about foods where gluten can hide may seem like a daunting task; however, when you realize your child's health is at stake, you know it is a venture you must undertake.

Depending upon the age of your child, eliminating gluten from their diet may prove to be quite a challenge. If breads, cereals, pastries, and pasta are a normal part of their daily eating, eliminating them or offering substitutions in their place will take some time and adjustments.

Also, consider the implications involved in this change in eating for your child. If you eliminate breads and pastas from your child's diet, yet they remain in your pantry for the rest of your family to enjoy, this could prove to create tension and become a difficult situation.

Because of the family dynamics involved in this type of scenario, many parents decide it is time to make permanent changes in the whole family's diet so their child does not feel ostracized or singled out because of food and health issues. Many have found that by doing this, it simplifies grocery shopping, food preparation, and often lowers the stress level of family members and restores harmony in the home.

At this point, there is a statistic that may help motivate you as you contemplate whether to try to change your whole family's diet to gluten-free. As many as 30% to 50% of the world's population are gluten-sensitive,[9] yet many people do not even realize they are. This means your whole family could benefit from eliminating gluten from their diets, even though they do not believe they have a gluten allergy.

As we have already discussed, some debilitating symptoms can manifest themselves in your child's physical and emotional conditions when they consume foods containing gluten. In this next section, I want to share with you reasons why eliminating gluten may also improve the health and well being of your child and the rest of your family members.

Gluten-containing grains are high in carbohydrates, resulting in your insulin levels elevating after you eat them. After you eat, you want your blood glucose to rise slowly and maintain a constant level. You do not want rapid rises that result in high peaks in your sugar levels. Ultimately, you want your glucose levels to rise slowly and fall gently as your body begins to warn you that you are hungry and telling you it is time to eat again. You never want to suddenly feel famished or shaky, yet a diet high in grains and carbohydrates can cause these things to happen.

All foods that affect your blood-sugar levels have been given a number on a scale called the Glycemic Index Foods List. This list consists of foods that physically affect the glucose levels in your blood. Foods that are low on the GI scale are ones like vegetables, nuts, and fruits. Foods that have a high GI score are foods like potatoes, rice, and breads. Though it may seem strange, whole grain breads are actually at the high end of the Glycemic Index.

To give you a frame of reference for what this scale indicates, eating pure glucose would have a glycemic index number of 100. This would be at the top end of the scale, resulting in a rapid rise in blood glucose and a high insulin response as well.

Along with the number scale, there are three main categories. Each category consists of how different foods affect our sugar levels.[10]

— The first category comprises low GI foods and they are
given a number of 0 through 55
— The second category is for medium GI foods that have
been assigned a number from 56 to 70
— And finally, the third category is the one for high GI
foods that are given a number from 70 to 100

To categorize some of the well-known carbohydrate foods, let me give you a few examples, followed by their number on the Glycemic Index scale. Be sure to notice how they range from lowest to highest:

— Bulgur wheat – 48
— Brown rice – 54
— Pita bread – 57
— Couscous – 65
— Whole wheat bread – 68
— Bagel – 72
— White bread – 79
— French bread – 95

As the numbers demonstrate, grains cause a rapid rise in blood sugar levels, resulting in a strong insulin release.

What is amazing to me is that all of these bread products have a higher glycemic index than eating plain table sugar, which is 50 on the GI scale! In reality, it is not the gluten in bread that causes the rise in blood sugar levels. That distinction goes to the grains themselves. However, decreasing grains that contain gluten will diminish the problems brought on with rapid changes in blood sugar.

Another problem associated with gluten-containing foods is the recently discovered fact that proteins within the gluten family can interact with the opiate receptors in your brain. Because gluten allergies and sensitivities can affect mental capabilities, parents of children with autism have been eliminating gluten-containing foods from their children's diets as one of the first steps toward improving their children's health.

You may have joked in the past that you were addicted to doughnuts but there is more reality to that claim than you might like to admit. Many people who start a low-carb diet usually eliminate grains from their diet right off the bat. Because of this, they often suffer what is known as "low-carb flu." This often lasts for several days early on in their diet as they deal with "carb withdrawal."

In his book, *The Paleo Solution*, author Robb Wolf humorously describes how hard it is to talk people into giving up gluten-filled grains from their diet. He says:

Not only do grains make you sick by raising insulin levels, messing up your fatty acid ratios and irritating your gut, but they are also addictive. Grains, particularly the gluten-containing grains, contain molecules that fit into the opiate receptors in our brain. You know, the same receptors that work with heroine, morphine, and Vicodin? Most people can take or leave stuff like corn tortillas and rice. [They don't contain gluten]. Suggest that people should perhaps forgo bread and pasta for their health and they will bury a butter knife in your forehead before you can say "whole wheat!"[11]

If you are still not completely sure that eliminating gluten from your child's diet—and even yours—is a good idea, try the advice of many who have gone before you:

— Begin by abstaining from eating any gluten for 30 days and see how you feel at the end of the time period

— Then, at the end of 30 days, try eating something with gluten in it and see what happens and how you feel

Like many who have done this (myself included), you may experience a complete disappearance of symptoms you thought you were destined to live with – symptoms like irritable bowel syndrome, eczema, headaches, and other ones we have discussed before. By doing so, you may feel as though something *magical* has happened in your life.

As has been the case with many people, you may feel better at the end of the 30 days than you ever thought possible. You may even find that for the first time in your life, your days are symptom-free.

While no one would say you should be thankful for your child having problems with gluten, it could actually prove to be a blessing on some levels. By eliminating gluten from your child's diet and even choosing to do the same thing yourself, you and your family may find they ultimately feel better than they ever have before. At the very least, it is worth doing it for the sake of your child!

Well, now that I have challenged you personally to not only eliminate gluten from your child's diet but also from the diet of your whole family, let me explain to you the differences between gluten-free and grain-free. Understanding the distinction between the two will enable you to have a better understanding of their terminology and what they involve.

CHAPTER 4:
How Does a Gluten-Free Diet Compare to a Grain-Free Diet?

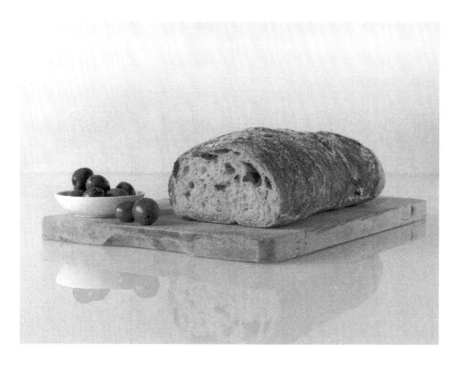

As I have discussed with you previously, gluten is a sticky protein found in many grains that are used in making pizza, breads, and pastries. However, gluten is not found in every grain. Therefore, a gluten-free diet means your child can consume some grains and other foods that do not have any gluten in them at all.

Grain free, on the other hand, is exactly what it means. A person does not include any grains at all in their diet. Therefore, if you were to decide to go grain free, that means you would no longer eat any grains at all – no wheat, rice, corn, barley – none! That may sound really difficult to do at first; however, as we go along, you may find that going gluten-free is just as difficult, if not harder to do than eliminating grains.

While gluten is present in some grains, it is not in others. If you are going to change your child's diet to "gluten free," it is possible for them to enjoy *some* grains but it will become necessary for both of you to learn which ones contain gluten and which ones do not. For examples, some grains that do not contain gluten are rice, buckwheat, teff, corn, and oat.

Grains such as spelt, wheat, kamut, rye, and barley are grains that do have gluten. Some have a higher percentage of gluten than others, but they all contain some amounts of gluten. This is a key difference between the two types of diets: people who choose to eat gluten-free can still eat some grains, but people who choose to eat grain-free end up eliminating grains totally from their diet.

Nowadays, people commonly eliminate grains from their diet because they want to cut down on carbohydrates, they want to lose weight, and they want to discover if they have any sensitivity to gluten. This approach tends to be more of a **choice** rather than a necessity. This type of diet has several different names like a Paleo diet, a Primal diet, the Caveman diet, and a Paleolithic diet to name a few.

By eliminating grains totally from their diet, Paleolithic eaters often experience signs of improved health because not only have they given up a huge percentage of carbohydrates they used to consume, but they also notice symptoms related to gluten sensitivities begin to disappear.

The bottom line between the two types of eating comes down to this: *Gluten-free means you can still eat some grains—grain-free means all grains are eliminated from your diet.* As a result, many have begun to adapt a grain-free diet as the safest and healthiest way to live a gluten-free diet because it totally eliminates the possibilities of cross-contamination.

In contrast to a grain-free diet, someone choosing to eat a gluten-free diet can still enjoy grains like oat, buckwheat, rice, and sorghum; however, it becomes necessary to use them in various combinations with other non-gluten flours and ingredients in order to make breads, pastas, and pizza crusts.

As you are learning which foods are safest for your child, realize that whenever you see the words, "wheat-free" on food labels, this does NOT necessarily mean "gluten-free." For instance, if barley or rye is used in place of a wheat ingredient, it does not mean it is gluten-free because both barley and rye contain gluten.

On a gluten-free diet, your child can still eat foods like rice, beans, and even gluten-free pastas and breads. You may have noticed how there are more and more products coming out on the market that claim to be "gluten-free" as they respond to this ever-growing problem among children and adults alike.

To conclude this section, both a gluten-free diet and a grain-free diet have some similarities and both are becoming easier to accomplish as products and information are becoming more readily available. Although this resource is not intended to argue one diet over another, I felt it was important for you to understand some of the differences and similarities between these two ways of eating. Whichever one you choose for your child, and maybe even yourself, research indicates you will be taking steps toward better health for you and your family.

In the next chapter, we are going to discuss how to begin making changes toward a gluten-free diet.

CHAPTER 5:
Where Do I Begin?

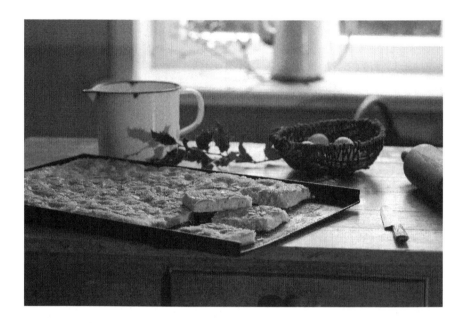

To start to comprehend some of what you will be dealing with in this lifestyle change, let me give you a short list of products. As you read or hear each one, decide whether or not it contains gluten. As you will discover, gluten can be found in some of the strangest places.

— Licorice

— Mouthwash

— Flavored potato chips

— Cosmetics

— Soy sauce

— Shampoos

— Chicken, and beef broth

— Lotions

— Teas like holiday and specialty flavors

— Beer

— Paints

— Dressings

— Play dough

— Marinades

— Soups

— Sunscreen

— Toothpaste

If you answered "yes" to every one of the items listed, you would have made a perfect score! It is rather amazing where gluten hides, isn't it?

Now here are some others that could be included in the list of foods that contain gluten:

— Orzo

— Panko bread crumbs

— Strudel

— Matzo

— Croutons

— Barley

— Bran

— Bulgur

— Rye

— Graham flour

— Durum

— Farina

— Ramen noodles

— Modified food starch

— Burritos

— Couscous

— Semolina

Realize this is by no means an exhaustive list! It is a big job learning what foods contain gluten and which ones do not. Fortunately, more and more information is becoming available as manufacturers and consumers find it necessary to address this health condition. Products labeled "gluten free" are coming into the marketplace as a way of helping consumers discover products that are safe for their dietary needs.

Gluten is being eliminated from the diets of those who are gluten-sensitive, gluten-intolerant, and those with celiac disease, but it is gaining popularity with people who do not have a "noticeable" problem eating it. Eliminating gluten has started becoming a choice many people are making in an effort to cut carbohydrates and for losing weight as well. There is some debate among the dietary community as to whether or not this is a good idea, but it is happening nonetheless.

In the beginning, you will want to focus on some main food categories as you make decisions concerning how to change the way your child eats. I think it will be easiest if we address some of them and break them down into smaller sections. Since breads are probably the biggest category to deal with, let us begin with this one.

Grains and Breads: When transitioning to a gluten-free diet, bread is something you can continue to eat; *however, now it must be gluten-free bread.* In the beginning, you will need to look extensively for gluten-free bread. This is easier than it used to be. The trick will be finding one that tastes good.

One thing you both will quickly discover is that gluten-free breads have a different texture and taste from breads you are used to. This may take some getting used to, so be patient with your child as they learn to make the switch.

Numerous gluten-free breads can be purchased at bigger grocery chains and specialty grocery stores. Start by checking the freezer section. Gluten-free breads are usually frozen so their shelf life can be extended. Like many other products, some of them are good while others taste like sawdust. You will have to experiment to see which ones your child enjoys. Fortunately, new breads are coming on the market all the time as manufacturers continue to try new combinations.

You might also try finding bread recipes on the Internet. More and more people have begun to share their recipe efforts with people on the Web as they work together to find "enjoyable alternatives" to whole-grain breads.

While you are trying to find breads your child likes, consider having them use lettuce, corn and brown rice tortillas for their sandwiches. Not only are these healthy alternatives, but they will buy you some time as you continue your search for new sandwich breads.

As you look for alternatives to wheat products, consider rice. Rice is a grain that is gluten free. Consider buying whole grain brown rice, as well as risotto, basmati, and jasmine rice.

If you purchase oats, make sure they do not contain gluten, especially if they are processed commercially. This is because cross contamination with other grains that do contain gluten can be a real danger in their processing. Find out if cross contamination occurs during harvesting, storing and milling. If oats are processed with other grains that contain gluten, do not risk it. There are manufacturers that offer oats that are certified gluten-free. Go with these and always look for "gluten-free" on the label.

Fruits and vegetables: Fortunately, all fruits and vegetables are free of gluten when they are eaten fresh. When you buy them in cans or from the freezer section, be sure to read the labels because any that contain sauces and other additives may have had gluten added. A good rule when starting out is to keep it simple and purchase fresh as much as possible.

Meats, Poultry, and Seafood: Red meats, pork, chicken, turkey, fish, and seafood are all naturally gluten-free. Problems arise when sauces, broths, seasonings and marinades are added to them. Whenever possible, feed your child fresh or plain frozen meats so you know what they are consuming.

Dairy: If your child does not have any problems with dairy, then this area will not require very many changes. Consider cultured plain organic yogurts instead of flavored ones. This allows you to add your own honey and gluten-free fruit jams if desired. Flavored yogurts may contain ingredients made with barley, and added granolas can cause gluten problems for your child.

When purchasing cheese, aged cheeses are safest because the lactose levels are almost zero after processing. As cheese ages, the lactose levels drop so these are the safest ones to consume. Just make sure to watch for any added flavorings in the cheeses you buy.

Some gluten-sensitive children also have problems with the casein, whey proteins, and lactose found in milk. Some will continue to have gluten-related symptoms even after they have had gluten eliminated from their diet. If this happens with your child, consider taking an additional step of eliminating milk proteins and lactose from their diet for 30 days to see if their symptoms improve or disappear. If so, take the next step of eliminating dairy as much as possible from their diet.

If you choose to purchase low-fat dairy products, be sure to read the labels for any added fillers and starches. Some of these may have gluten in them. Consider purchasing gluten-free vegan cheese alternatives that are made from almonds and rice. Start with labels that say "gluten-free" on the packaging and go from there. Be sure to call the manufacturers if you have questions. Also, be sure you learn the derivative names for casein, whey and lactose so you will know what you are purchasing.

In the Category of Miscellaneous Foods:

— Most **tofu** is gluten-free. Read the labels carefully and watch out for varieties of tofu that contain flavorings

— **Seitan** is made from vital wheat gluten so you definitely want to avoid purchasing this product for your child

— **Potatoes** are all gluten-free. However, if you buy them already processed, be sure and read the labels for any additives in the sauces or flavorings

— **Polenta** is made from cornmeal and should say "gluten free" on the packaging to ensure that it is safe enough for your child to eat

Foods to Avoid

When striving to eat a gluten-free diet, you will find yourself evaluating *everything* your child eats. Because your child's intestines have been inflamed and damaged over time, you will want to avoid some foods as you help your child on the road to recovery.

— First, avoid processed foods, junk foods, fast foods, and pre-packaged snack foods as much as possible. It is easy for food to become cross-contaminated in restaurants and packaging plants unless they are totally dedicated to being gluten free. We will discuss more about how to eat out safely in a later chapter

— Next, be sure to read the labels on **herbal teas and tea blends**, especially if your child enjoys drinking iced tea. Some of these have flavors and additives that contain malt and barley. Depending upon the age of your child, this may not concern you immediately

— Sugar alcohols often found in processed foods, drinks, and diet foods can negatively affect your child's digestive system by causing bloating, gas pains, and even diarrhea. Do your best to have your child eat organic and raw sugars that are not highly processed

Now that we have talked about purchasing food and others to avoid, you will need to learn some of the different names used for wheat in foods. Knowing them will help you recognize potential dangers of additives in food products so your child does not consume gluten by mistake.

To begin, avoid any food products that have the word "wheat" in them. These include ingredients like wheat germ and starch, as well as hydrolyzed wheat protein. One exception to this rule is wheat grass. Just as the name indicates, it is a grass and is gluten-free.

When a product claims to be "wheat-free," this does not mean it is gluten-free. Some ingredient names and products you will want to avoid are the following. As I begin, some have been mentioned before, but they are worth repeating:

— Malt

— Cake flour

— Kamut

— Bulgur

— Triticale

— Flour

— Couscous

— Matzah

— Semolina

— Durum

— Graham

— Seitan

— Einkorn

— Farina

— Spelt

— Matzo, and

— Frumento

While this is not an exhaustive list of foods to avoid, it is very important for you to learn terminology, read product labels, deal with dairy products, and memorize derivative names for wheat.

In this chapter, we have dealt with becoming familiar with labeling and terminology. Next, we will talk about how this knowledge will help you deal with food items you currently have in your home.

CHAPTER 6:
What Will My Pantry and Refrigerator Look Like without Gluten?

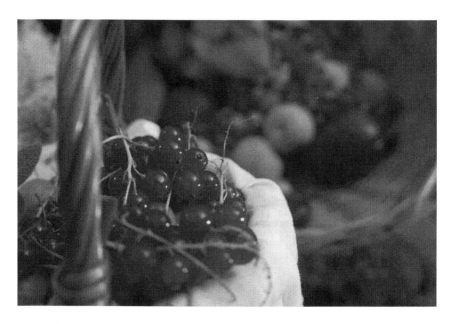

Another step in this process is for you to know which foods you have at home are okay for your child to eat and which ones you need to toss. Again, you need to be familiar with terminology and you must read each food label in your refrigerator and pantry cabinets carefully.

If any of the items you currently have in the house contain gluten of any kind and they are unopened, consider giving the items to your friends who can eat gluten, your local food bank or other charitable organizations. If others have already been opened, empty the contents and recycle the container if recycling is available in your area.

Some items are ones you are not sure about because you may not have had time to research whether or not the added ingredients contain gluten. In this case, put them aside so you can look them up later.

Once you have gone through all the food items in your home, you are ready to tackle the grocery store. This is the topic we will discuss in the next chapter.

Before we leave this section, there is one other area to touch upon. If you discover your child has a severe case of gluten sensitivity or has been diagnosed with celiac disease, you may need to deal with tougher issues like removing old cutting boards, repainting the walls in your kitchen, cleaning handles and knobs, and wiping down countertops with disinfectants. Vacuuming, wiping, scrubbing, and scraping can be quite laborious for removing gluten particles in the beginning, but once these things are accomplished, life can begin to get back to some form of normalcy.

Remember: give yourself time! It is a huge task to go through everything you have stored in your refrigerator and pantry cabinets and to de-contaminate your working space. Be realistic with your expectations and tackle each job one at a time.

CHAPTER 7:
What Does a Gluten-Free Shopping List Look Like?

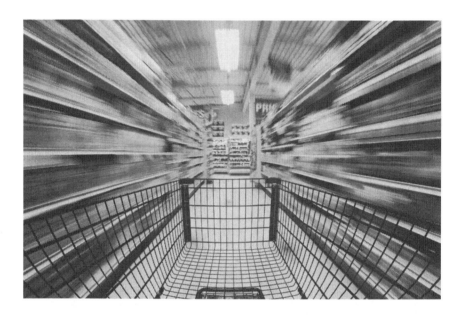

Your first trip to the grocery store can prove to be overwhelming. Reading labels and the fine print on all the packaging can take hours when you are exploring a completely new way of eating and cooking. Before you tackle the store, develop a plan that will work for you. Come up with your own personal strategy.

A good way to start is to list your normal menu recipes. Then look at each ingredient and substitute out the ones that contain gluten with ones that do not. For instance, if you enjoy cooking stir-fry for your child, feel free to continue to do so, but use gluten-free soy sauce instead.

One of the biggest areas you will need to change is pastas and breads. Now you will have to find pasta products that say "gluten-free" or substitute rice and even spaghetti squash in its place.

You will also have to experiment with different brands and types of sandwich breads until you find ones your child likes. As we discussed earlier, these are usually found in the freezer section of your grocery store or at your local health food store.

Next, eliminate grains and wheat dishes that have gluten in them and become familiar with the alternatives available to you. There are several gluten-free grains and flours you can use in your cooking that are safe for your child to eat. You can find many of them at larger grocery stores and even online.

This next section gives you some names of non-gluten grains and flours you can use in your cooking. When time allows, you can come back to this list as you make substitutions.

Millet flour: You can buy millet seeds and make your own flour using a high-speed blender. It is a good source of protein, B-complex, lecithin, magnesium, and potassium.

Brown rice flour: This whole grain is used to replace wheat flour and is often part of a gluten-free all-purpose baking mix. It is high in protein, fiber, and B vitamins.

Sweet rice flour: This makes a nice addition to baking mixes that are used for breads and pizzas.

Amaranth flour: This flour is used in combination with other flours for baking. It is high in protein, fiber, zinc, calcium and iron.

Sorghum flour: In recipes, it replaces wheat flour and adds a great texture to baked goods. It is high in antioxidants, fiber, iron, and protein.

Quinoa flour and flakes: This grain is used for making muffins, breads, and cookies. Some enjoy substituting quinoa for oatmeal. It is a complete protein containing calcium, fiber, manganese, copper, and magnesium and gives baked goods a nutty taste.

Buckwheat flour and groats: This nutritious grain has a distinctive flavor often used in soups, cereals, waffles, and pancakes. It is high in fiber, B vitamins and lysine, and is rich in other vitamins like copper, iron, manganese, and magnesium.

Teff flour: A grain high in nutrients, it contains iron, calcium, vitamin C, fiber and thiamin and also adds moistness to baked goods.

Almond flour and almond meal: A highly nutritious flour made from almonds, it is easy to find and to use. It is low in carbs and sugars, but is high in protein and is often used for making crusts.

Coconut flour: A flour made from the meat of the coconut, it has many nutrients, is a great source of fiber, and adds moisture to baked goods.

Corn flour and corn meal: Corn flour is ground finer than corn meal. Look for "whole" and "not degermed" on the product label to ensure it has not been genetically modified. Rich in fiber and antioxidants, corn meal and corn flour add a nutty taste to baked goods.

Oat flour: A flour high in minerals and fiber, be sure to look for labeling that promises no cross-contamination with other grains.

Because these flours do not contain any gluten, they have to be combined with other flours and ingredients to make baked goods. There are now many helpful resources and cookbooks on the market that can help you learn how to cook with them.

Now that you have a better idea of the types of flours that are safe for a gluten-free diet, I want to give you a few more tips on how to adapt your grocery shopping.

— First, whenever you buy flour and ready-made meals, try to purchase products with labels that use terms like "organic, gluten-free, whole grain, and all-natural."

— Next, start your grocery list with items you are familiar with and concentrate on buying them first. An example would be to purchase fresh fruits, vegetables, and meats to use in your cooking and as snacks. This will give you time to continue your studies on this topic so you can learn about other safe alternatives

— Be sure to keep track of items you buy on a regular basis by listing them on your computer or smartphone. Draw a map of the layout of your favorite grocery store and arrange your items in the order you come to them when you shop. While this takes some time in the beginning, it will save you time later on

— If you see an item you think is promising but are not sure of some of its ingredients, write down the ingredients and look them up at home. Additionally, you can take a picture of the ingredients with your smartphone and research them later

— Finally, keep track of brand-name foods that are gluten-free by writing down ones you have read about on the Internet or have learned about from magazines, books and friends.

Nowadays, many products that are processed and labeled "gluten free" help make shopping easier. However, if you are not sure and if you are not familiar with a particular product, be sure to read the product's label carefully before purchasing it. You can also contact the manufacturer to see if a product is processed in a plant where cross contamination occurs. There is usually a phone number listed on the product that you can call to make sure the product is safe for you to buy for your child. If it is not labeled or you are not sure, do not buy it!

Fortunately, many items you already eat are ones that do not have gluten in them so it may not be as difficult for you to begin this process as you may have initially thought.

In this section, I want to provide you with some items for your shopping list that have been shown to be safe and gluten-free. If you would like a list of them so you can print them out and take the list to the grocery store, you will find a PDF file at UnitedPublishingHouse.com listed under the title of this book (http://unitedpublishinghouse.com/products/gluten-free-kids/).

For the sake of time and space, I will give you a few examples from each of the main food categories. For a more thorough listing, once again the PDF can be found at UnitedPublishingHouse.com (http://unitedpublishinghouse.com/products/gluten-free-kids/).

A Gluten-Free Shopping List

Under the category of grains, pastas, cereals, and chips, the following are gluten-free and safe to purchase:

— Arrowroot starch

— Crackers made from corn, lentils, and brown rice varieties but make sure they are labeled gluten free

— Dry cereal varieties made with corn, rice, amaranth, millet, buckwheat, and soy

— Pastas made from brown rice, corn, peas, beans, potatoes, lentils, soy, or quinoa

— Plain corn chips

— Popcorn. Air-popped popcorn varieties and packages labeled gluten-free are best

— Rice varieties that are wild, brown, basmati, and risotto

— Rice cakes that are plain are the safest

— Taco shells made from corn

— Tortilla chips that are plain are safest

Under the category of dairy, here are some guidelines to follow:

The low-fat varieties and the reduced fat cheeses are good to start with.

— Aged cheeses are best if you suspect dairy is an issue

— Cottage cheeses

— Cream cheeses

— When considering ice cream, be sure to read the labels for each flavor

— Milk

— Milk alternatives such as rice, soy, and almond

— Plain yogurts and

— Sour creams

When it comes to buying fruits:

— All fresh fruits are gluten free. If you buy frozen fruits, be sure to check the label for any added ingredients

When purchasing vegetables and legumes:

— All fresh vegetables and frozen vegetables that do not have any added breading, additives, or sauces are safe. Be sure to read the packaging before buying any

— Canned beans are gluten-free

— All fresh varieties of potatoes are gluten-free. If buying canned or frozen, be sure to read the labels

In the category of meats, poultry, seafood and other proteins:

— All fresh meats, poultry, shellfish, and fish are gluten-free. If buying frozen or canned, be sure to check for additives such as breading

— Eggs are fine

— Plain tofu is best. Read labels if you wish to purchase flavored tofu

For the category of nuts and seeds:

— All nuts, nut butters, and seeds are fine

If using oils:

— Purchase coconut oil, olive oil, and nut oils

In the category of vinegars:

— Purchase apple cider, red wine, white wine, white, or balsamic

With herbs and spices,

— All **pure** herbs and spices are gluten-free. If you want to purchase herb and spice mixes, be sure to read the labels

In the area of baking goods and condiments, there are many to choose from. Some you are certainly familiar with like:

— Baking chocolate

— Baking powder

— Baking soda

— Cocoa powder

— Instant and ground coffees are fine. Be sure to check the ingredients of flavored coffees

— Extracts like vanilla, rum, and almond

— Garlic

— Honey

— Ketchup

— Mustard

— Pickles

— Salsa

— Sugar and

— Black and green teas. Be sure to read the labels on flavored teas

When desiring to use sweeteners, focus on natural sugars like

— Raw honey

— Blackstrap molasses and

— Pure maple syrup

From a health standpoint, try to eat the freshest and purest products you can afford. However, whenever you buy packaged or processed foods, be sure to read the labeling, which I know can be quite confusing.

To close out this section on grocery shopping, I want to share with you a list of additives that gluten-free. Although I am only going to share a few with you here, once again you can consult the PDF for a gluten-free shopping list at UnitedPublishingHouse.com (http://unitedpublishinghouse.com/products/gluten-free-kids/)[12]

— Arrowroot

— Ascorbic acid

— Aspic

— BHA

— BTA

— Dextrose

— Fructose

— Guar gum

— Locust bean gum

— Malic acid

— Pectin

— Pepsin

— Sulfites

— Tapioca starch and flour

— Whey, and

— Xanthan gum

Now that you have been working hard to learn and process the information and changes involved in switching to a gluten-free diet, it is time to talk about how to discuss these changes with your child. This is what will be discussed in the next chapter.

CHAPTER 8:
How Do I Talk to My Child about Gluten Sensitivity?

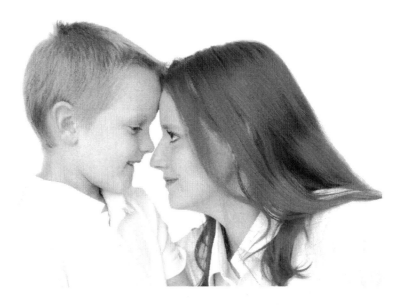

Eventually, you will have to talk with your child about their medical condition. Some of this will be determined by the age of your child and by the urgency of the situation.

At some point when you determine the time is right, it will be necessary for you to help your child understand the types of foods that are safe for him to eat and ones he will need to learn to avoid. This is especially important if your child is in school and away from you at different times of the day. Being patient with your child, explaining his condition to him, and allowing your child to ask questions are extremely important aspects involved in discussions about his health.

As you consider how to approach this subject with your child, let me offer some of the following suggestions to help you. Even if you have already spoken to your child about their condition, you may find some additional suggestions helpful as your child ages and to offer further explanations that are more thorough. In reality, this will be a discussion you will not want to have with your child until you have a good grasp of the information yourself.

Begin by talking with your child about how they have been feeling physically. Whether it is vomiting, cramping, headaches, or bloating, start by discussing how your child has been feeling.

Next, talk together about how certain foods make him feel after he eats them. Keep a food journal together. Let your child share with you how he feels physically after eating foods like fruits, bagels, salads, and pizza.

Help her understand what gluten is and which foods contain it. You may be able to find visual resources online or other materials at your local library that will provide explanations and pictures. These will explain what your child's body looks like internally and how gluten affects them. Make a game out of this. Buy some flashcards at your local school supply store or make your own as you teach your child which foods are good for them and which ones they need to avoid.

Explain to your child that gluten allergies and celiac disease affects many people. Because gluten negatively affects 1% of the American population, you can reassure your child that gluten intolerance is nothing to be ashamed of. Many food companies, restaurants, and other manufacturers are helping people with gluten sensitivities by offering healthy alternatives to their favorite foods.

Take them grocery shopping with you. This is a great way for your child to acquire some hands-on learning. You could use this as a time of testing after the two of you have studied about gluten-containing foods. This would also be a great time to offer a reward like going some place special or money if they pass the test! In addition, depending upon the age of your child, you can show them how to read various food labels and what ingredients to avoid.

Cook together. When you cook together, you can demonstrate how to substitute delicious, non-gluten foods for ones he used to eat. For example, explain how cooking from scratch is a safer way to cook because you know what is in your food. Also, show him how foods like spaghetti squash can be eaten in place of pasta. Make this time one of fun and experimentation.

Teach your child how to politely explain their condition to others. Practice with your child what they should say to their teachers, extended family members, and friends concerning their medical condition. Help them practice saying it in a positive way, too. A simple statement like, "I cannot eat foods with wheat, rye, or barley because they make me sick," is a helpful way to alert others who may have responsibility for the care of your child when you are apart from each other.

Have fun throwing a party for your child's friends. Invite your child's friends and their parents over for a gluten-free party. Not only will this educate others, but it will also demonstrate that eating gluten-free can be fun.

Expect your child to eat gluten on occasion. Part of the "learning curve" involved in raising a child with gluten sensitivities is expecting them to try foods they have learned are not good for them. Whether it is peer pressure or just curiosity, at some point your child will try foods he knows he should not eat. In most situations, the consequences of how he feels after doing so will be his best teacher. Ultimately, his body's reactions to gluten-laden foods are enough to keep him on his diet in the future.

I hope this chapter has helped you figure out how to discuss your child's medical condition with them. Now, let us explore some meal and snack ideas you can enjoy together.

CHAPTER 9:
What Do Meals and Snacks Look Like for My Child?

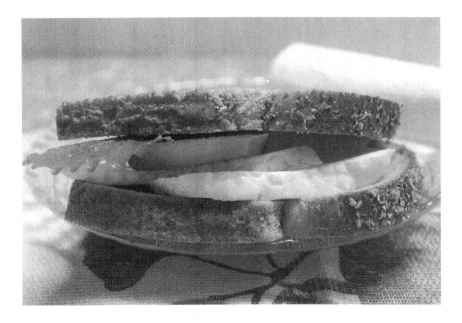

As you begin to understand the changes involved in providing a gluten-free diet for your child, I thought it would be helpful to give you some practical ideas of what snacks and mealtimes could look like. These are some examples to help you see there are many foods available to you as you get your creative juices flowing. As you become even more knowledgeable about this form of eating, you will enjoy even more variety in your eating.

You can find other ideas and resources on the Internet as more and more people have started sharing their experiences, information, recipe ideas and food choices that can be found in the marketplace.

Here are some gluten-free snack ideas:

— Apple slices with a chunk of aged cheddar cheese

— Salads with almonds, pecans, and walnuts added

— Fresh grapes with a slice of aged cheddar cheese

— Flavored yogurt using plain cultured organic yogurt and natural fruit preserves. Use preserves that are low in sugar or ones that are labeled "no sugar added"

— Banana slices with fresh-ground peanut butter on a corn tortilla

— Baby carrots or carrot sticks dipped in your favorite salsa or gluten-free dip

— Trail mix with dried apples, raisins, and nuts

— Gluten-free corn tortilla chips with your favorite salsa or homemade guacamole dip

— Rice cakes spread with natural nut butters. Add a little bit of raw honey if you like

— There are gluten-free *goodies* you can buy such as ice cream and sorbets, popsicles and fruit bars. Gluten-free baked goods are available for purchase as well

How about some gluten-free mealtime ideas to try:

— Stir-fry is a great way to eat healthy and gluten-free. Cut up a bunch of fresh vegetables or thawed frozen vegetables without added flavorings and sauces, add some meat strips like beef or chicken, and flavor it with gluten-free sauces

— Have a baked potato night. Cook up whole white potatoes or sweet potatoes and enjoy adding vegetables, homemade meat sauces and chilies that you know are gluten-free. Top with some aged shredded cheeses for a great-tasting meal

— Soups and stews for lunch and dinner are great choices, too

— Use different types of rice with your stir-fry and sauces

— Lunches can be similar to dinners by having salads that contain meat strips, nuts, dried and fresh fruits

— Breakfast time gives possibilities for egg dishes like frittatas and omelets that contain onions, mushrooms, bell peppers and aged cheeses

— Look for cereals that are labeled "gluten-free" and enjoy them with almond or rice milk. Be sure to read the labels to make sure they are gluten free

— Gluten-free waffles are readily available for purchase. Top them with fresh fruit or pure maple syrup

— Quinoa, millet, and rice can be cooked to make a hearty breakfast cereal you can top with cinnamon, raw honey or pure maple syrup and nuts

— Smoothies made with plain cultured yogurt, frozen fruits and honey are a delicious way to start the day

Remember that all vegetables and fruits are gluten free, as are meats, poultry, pork, fish and seafood as long as they have not been processed with added sauces and flavorings that contain gluten products.

Think healthy when you start to think of ways to serve snacks and meals for your family. As you can imagine, eating a gluten-free diet can be a way to bring more fruits, meats, and vegetables into your child's diet.

So what does your child's school lunch look like when gluten is not an option? Well, this just happens to be what we will talk about in the next chapter.

CHAPTER 10:
How Do I Deal with School Lunches?

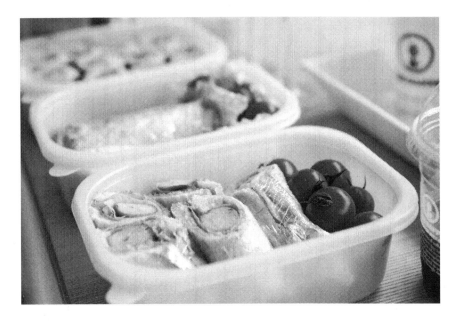

Depending upon the severity of your child's medical condition, you may have difficulty figuring out which foods to send with him to school. Maybe the difficulty is not necessarily in having choices, but rather in helping your child keep a good attitude about having to eat foods other than what their classmates are eating.

As you think through options of what to include in your child's lunchbox, here are a few tips on how to help your child have a positive attitude about their lunch options.

First, involve your child in the process. As the two of you are forced to make changes, approach it like an adventure. Ask your child what kinds of food she has seen other children bring for lunch that she might like to have as well. Take those items and try to figure out substitutions or find gluten-free options.

Plan a week's worth of lunches together. Have your child help you pack their lunches. Getting your child involved will help them take ownership and often get them excited about the choices they have been allowed to make.

Purchase a lunchbox and a thermos that can keep foods cold and hot. With your child's involvement, explore various lunchboxes that allow foods to remain cold. This will give you opportunities to pack deli meats, salads and dressings, and other items that need to maintain some type of refrigeration. In addition, having a thermos that can keep foods hot gives you options for sending soups to school on chilly days.

Focus on proteins, fruits, and vegetables. As you plan your child's lunches with them, encourage them to choose foods like fresh fruits, salads, cheeses, and deli meats on a regular basis. Because gluten-free foods sometimes lack minerals and vitamins, it is important to focus on foods that are known for their health benefits.

Offer treats in their lunchbox. Take time to ask your child what they consider treats. Whether it is gluten-free cookies or candies that are safe for him to eat, stock up on these items and allow them to include them in their lunches. This often gives them something to look forward to and can keep them from wishing they had someone else's lunch instead.

Speak with your child's teachers. Because your child will be away from you during school hours, it is important to make your child's teachers aware of his allergies. This will help the teachers, not only on a daily basis, but when special parties or events are planned for the class. Think about putting a laminated list in your child's lunchbox or school notebooks for easy reference.

Talk with your child about not exchanging food. It is especially important to stress to your child that they should not exchange food with their friends during lunchtime. Depending upon the age of your child, you may want to enlist the help from your child's teachers on this one.

To close out this section, I thought it might be helpful to give you some school lunch ideas you and your child could pack.

— Deviled eggs or hard boiled eggs

— Salads

— Tuna salad and chicken salad with gluten-free sandwich bread

— Applesauce

— Fresh fruit cups

— Sliced cucumbers with Italian dressing

— Carrot chips with dressing

— Homemade muffins

— Gluten-free Rice Krispies Treats

— String cheese with apple slices

— Chex mixes

— Popcorn

— Gluten-free pasta salads

— Homemade soups

— Leftover gluten-free pizza

— Veggie burgers

— Homemade chicken nuggets

— Dried fruits

— Trail mix made at home

— Mixed nuts with pumpkin seeds and sunflower seeds

— Jello cups

I hope this short list gives you some guidance and helpful lunch ideas as you and your child work together to deal with school lunches and the challenges they present. In the next chapter, we will tackle another area of concern— eating out in restaurants.

CHAPTER 11:
How Do We Eat Out Safely?

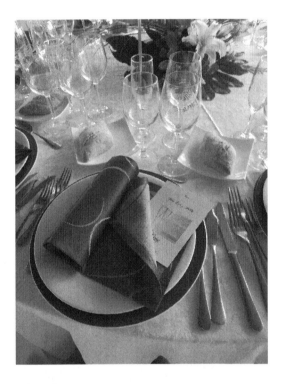

When your child suffers from gluten allergies, it can be difficult to find restaurants that offer options for a gluten-free diet. Initially, you may feel as though it is safest to always have them eat at home, especially when you are first making changes in their diet. This may actually prove to be the best idea while you give yourself time to learn what you need to know, what to look for, and the questions you will need to ask when dining out.

As more and more people become aware of gluten allergies, many restaurants and restaurant chains are trying to meet their needs. This makes dining out easier for families to do, as well as helping them feel safer. However, there are still numerous challenges involved when trying to maintain a gluten-free lifestyle.

For starters, many regional and national restaurant chains have started offering gluten-free menu items, as well as some fast-food chains. Knowing what to look for and how to ask questions about each business' food preparations are a big part of the safety and enjoyment concerning your child's eating experience. Here are some basic guidelines to help you knowledgeably tackle this area:

Start your research by searching online for eateries in your area that offer gluten-free options for children. Once you discover some, consider calling the restaurant ahead of time before you visit to inquire about their menu. Ask if they have any policies about bringing food items into their establishment for children with allergies.

Once you arrive, ask questions of the manager and specifically the chef because they will have had training concerning this issue. While you may be tempted to question the server, they usually are not as familiar with food preparations as the manager and chef are.

Next, check with the restaurant to see if they have a dedicated fryer for gluten-free frying. If your child likes fried foods, be sure to ask this question. Potatoes fried in the same fryer as battered onion rings are going to give your child problems with gluten.

If you think your child will want something ordered from the grill, check to see if marinades with gluten have been used on it. Marinades used for flavoring and thickening often contain gluten, so check with the manager to see if this will affect the items your child will want to order.

Realize there can be a real problem with cross-contamination. According to chef Kendall Egan, "Flour particles can take three days to settle. If a kitchen is making their own bread or dough and it is a shared kitchen, then it's more of a challenge. Not many kitchens have a separate pastry kitchen."[13]

When in doubt, ask questions. When ordering food for your child, be sure to ask how the food will be prepared to eliminate possibilities of cross contamination. When your child's food arrives at your table, oftentimes the manager will accompany the order; however, if not, be sure to ask the server questions of how it was prepared and to make sure it is exactly what was ordered and how you ordered it. Ultimately, if you are not satisfied with the results, **do not let your child eat it.**

Although it may prove awkward to receive the meal but not allow your child to eat it, it is certainly better for them to go hungry for a little while rather than suffer the consequences of a meal gone awry.

Finally, do not allow your child to eat off your plate or the plates of other family members. While your child's plate may have been prepared properly and be gluten-free, yours may not be. Avoid possible problems with gluten by having your child only eat from their own plate.

Learning to feel confident about eating out may take some time. Consult another friend or parent who is familiar with gluten-free cooking and ask them to accompany you and your child for an outing. Having two sets of ears and other people thinking along the same wavelength as you can diminish a lot of the stress involved in learning how to eat out successfully and enjoying the experience when first starting out.

In the next section, I want to share with you some of the latest findings concerning the link between gluten, ADD/ADHD and other problems children experience neurologically.

CHAPTER 12:
Is There a Link between Gluten, ADHD and Other Neurological Problems?

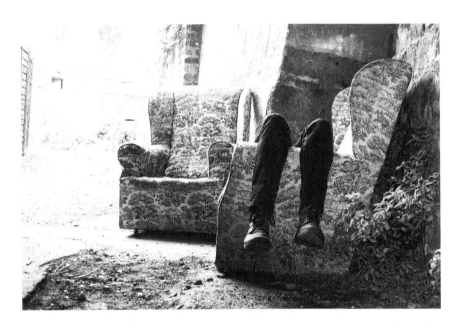

As we have talked about previously, there is an estimated one out of 133 people in the United States that have been diagnosed with celiac disease; however, the numbers may be as high as one out of 33 people who are at risk that suffer with some form of gluten sensitivity. Because this number is so high, more and more research has been occurring to study the implications of our dietary habits.

There is evidence suggesting that gluten sensitivity may be the root of many neurological and psychiatric conditions, including attention deficit hyperactivity disorder, otherwise known as ADHD.[14] In fact, "there may be a closer link between the symptoms of celiac disease and ADHD than was previously recognized, and that connection is gluten."[15]

Because there has been such a large increase in the number of children diagnosed with ADD and ADHD over the last few decades, and the growing amount of research that is beginning to link ADD and ADHD with gluten sensitivities, I wanted to focus your attention briefly on some of the symptoms involved in this area.

Before a child is diagnosed with ADD/ADHD, he must exhibit eight of the following fourteen signs:

1. Often talks excessively

2. Easily distracted

3. Has difficulty following instructions

4. Does not listen to what is being said

5. Easily forgets what is necessary for activities and tasks

6. Has problems with quiet play

7. Has problems with taking turns in group activities or playing games

8. Finds it difficult to remain seated when told to do so

9. Is fidgety with their hands and feet and is very wiggly when seated

10. Finds it difficult to follow instructions

11. Will take harmful physical risks without considering the possibilities of harmful consequences

12. Will interrupt or disturb others

13. Jumps from one task to another without completing any

14. Will blurt out answers before someone has finished asking the questions

If you believe your child exhibits many of the signs listed above, you may find this next section especially helpful.

In medicine, there is a principle known as the "gut-brain connection," stating the evidence that demonstrates there is gastrointestinal involvement found in numerous diseases involving the brain. In fact, Dr. Mercola states on his website that in essence we have two "brains" in our bodies—one in our head and one in our gut, and as such, they both require healthy nourishment. In large part, this is because during our development in the womb, our brain and intestinal tract are created out of the same tissue type, ultimately joined together by way of the tenth cranial nerve that extends from your brain stem down to your stomach.[16]

As a result, harmful and toxic substances in your intestines can circulate throughout your system and end up in your brain where it can result in symptoms of ADHD, schizophrenia, autism, depression, dyslexia, and other disorders of the brain.[17] Physiologically, most children that develop disorders such as these also have an inflammatory bowel condition as well. In addition, more than half of those who suffer with celiac disease also have problems neurologically.[18] This is why a gluten-free diet is so highly recommended.

Some who study nutrition recommend eliminating grains altogether so there is no chance of your child being affected by gluten. When living on a gluten-free diet, many depend upon food labeling as a way of feeling reassured that the foods their child is consuming are safe. However, when grains remain in your child's diet, depending solely upon gluten-free-labeling can even cause problems. One study tested 22 different products labeled "gluten-free," yet seven of them did not pass the standards set forth by the FDA.[19] This is another good reason for creating a diet for your child that is mostly whole foods.

Because there is such a strong correlation between diet and the treatment of ADHD and other mental disorders, here are some recommended steps you can take as a parent:

1. Avoid processed foods. So many processed foods contain preservatives, artificial colors, high fructose corn syrup, fructose, and artificial flavors that eliminating these from your child's diet can help relieve symptoms because gluten often hides in these products.

2. Eliminate grains and sugars. While eliminating gluten will often show improvement in your child's symptoms, totally eliminating grains is recommended as well to see if your child has even further improvement in his symptoms. In addition, sugars can often aggravate a child with allergies and gluten sensitivity so limit their intake of sugars as much as possible.

3. Increase your child's intake of Omega-3 fats. Make sure these are animal based and are a high quality supplement.

4. Increase your child's intake of lean protein, vegetables and whole fruits.

5. Eliminate soft drinks and fruit juices. Encourage your child to drink more water.

Keeping your child on a gluten-free diet is no easy task and if he "cheats" even a little bit, much of the progress you have made could be undone. While some symptoms of gluten sensitivity may improve quickly, others can take as long as a year before the lining of your child's intestinal tract is fully healed. This means it will be necessary for your child to follow a gluten-free diet for a long time before most of their symptoms lessen or disappear.

In Closing

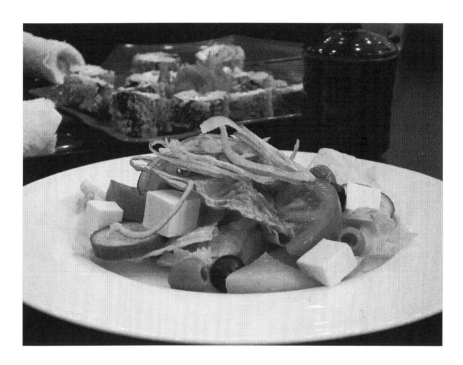

When your child is diagnosed with gluten allergies or celiac disease, eating and living gluten free becomes a completely new way of life. Plus, any time something as big as changing the way your child and your family eats, how you shop for food, products you cook with, and how you live your life are going to take **time.**

One of the biggest challenges involved in making major changes in your child's eating habits is giving yourself the time to get educated about foods that contain gluten and which ones do not, what needs to change in your home to keep gluten from re-entering it, and how to enjoy taking your child out to a restaurant.

As you have learned from the material presented here, there are many layers to this issue. I encourage you to consider finding a support group online, one that is located near you, or establish a closer relationship with the parents of other children with gluten allergies so you can lean on others as you work to gain understanding and help.

In addition, try to keep a positive attitude about your child's health issues and changes that must be made. Think of them as a new adventure in your life and of your child; one that offers new chances to learn, opportunities for changes, and the ultimate goal – a chance for your child to feel the best they have ever felt.

If your child has been suffering from gluten-related symptoms and you are finally on the road to eliminating health problem from their diet and life, you will begin to see them:

— Be more energetic

— Process situations better

— Concentrate for longer periods of time

— Experience a much better attitude

— And as their parent, you know these changes make all the hard work worth it!

For more information on celiac disease and dealing with children who have gluten allergies and sensitivities, check out organizations on the Internet such as:

— The Celiac Disease Awareness Campaign

http://celiac.nih.gov/

— The Gluten-Free Certification Organization

http://www.gfco.org/

— The Celiac Disease Foundation

http://www.celiac.org/

— CDF Resource Directory.com

http://glutenfreeresourcedirectory.com/uid/4df6c6a2

-2750-4966-a17d-540b30b115c5/

— The Gluten Intolerance Group of North America

http://www.gluten.net/

— and a wealth of information at Celiac.com

http://www.celiac.com/

Additional Resources

Additional works by Jennifer Wells

Going Gluten Free:
A Quick Start Guide for a Gluten-Free Diet

Juice for Health:
The Benefits of Juicing for Health and Wellness

Top 10 Tips to Help You Lose Weight

######

Acknowledgements

Many thanks to the following photographers for the use of their artwork in this eBook.

— Whatsername?

— Flyinace2000

— dailylifeofmojo

— jurvetson

— makelessnoise

— smith_cl9

— Rafael Tovar

— twid

— youngthousands

— MStewartPhotography

— Ali Brohi

— KayOne73

— Bunches and Bits (Karina)

— Patrick Hoesly

— juhansonin

About the Author

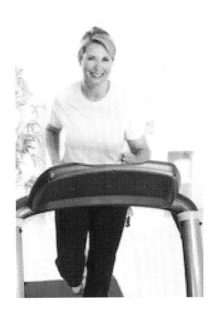

Always into sports and very active growing up, Jennifer never gave much thought to diet and exercise. Weight gain was not much of an issue. Then, after marriage and the birth of her twin boys, Jennifer noticed she had problems keeping her weight under control.

After numerous years of frustration, trying to get rid of stubborn pounds and not feeling as well as she wanted, Jennifer began her own personal research into diet and exercise. As a result, she ended up going back to school to get a degree in nutritional science.

Now she enjoys living a healthy lifestyle, spending time outdoors, teaching classes on nutrition at her local high school, and sharing healthy tips and information with family and friends.

And just in case you are curious, Jennifer is now back down to her weight before she had her four children.

Endnotes

[1] Michelle Matte, *Gluten Sensitivity in Children,* September 4, 2011. Viewed online at http://www.livestrong.com/article/535058-gluten-sensitivity-in-children/ on 12.05.12.

[2] Ibid.

[3] Ibid.

[4] Dr. Rodney Ford, "Oats—Safe to Eat?" Viewed online at http://drrodneyford.com/extra/documents/234-oats-safe-to-eat.html on 12.05.12.

[5] "Coeliac Disease." Viewed online at http://en.wikipedia.org/wiki/Coeliac_disease on 09.12.12.

[6] Anna Wilde, "Gluten Intolerance Symptoms—How Do You Know If Gluten Is Making You Sick?" Viewed online at http://glutenfreenetwork.com/faqs/symptoms-treatments/gluten-intolerance-symptoms-how-do-you-know-if-gluten-is-making-you-sick/ on 12.05.12.

[7] Dr. Mercola, "Child Have ADHD? Stop Feeding Them This," November 2, 2011. Viewed online at http://articles.mercola.com/sites/articles/archive/2011/11/02/gluten-contribute-to-adhd.aspx on 12.13.12.

[8] Karen Plumley, "Signs & Symptoms of a Gluten Allergy in Kids." Viewed online at http://www.ehow.com/about_5084117_signs-symptoms-gluten-allergy-kids.html on 12.05.12.

[9] Jane Anderson, "How Many People Have Gluten Sensitivity?" February 26, 2012. Viewed online at http://celiacdisease.about.com/od/glutenintolerance/a/How-Many-People-Have-Gluten-Sensitivity.htm on 12.05.12.

[10] Glycemic Index List of Foods. Viewed online at http://www.lowgihealth.com.au/category/what-is-glycemic-index/ on 09.08.12.

[11] Robb Wolf, *The Paleo Solution Diet* (Las Vegas, NV: Victory Belt Publishing, 2010), 97.

[12] "The Ultimate Grocery List for Celiac Disease." Viewed online at http://www.joybauer.com/celiac/food-list.aspx on 09.07.12.

[13] Kendall Egan, "How Restaurant Kitchens Really Work." *Gluten-Free Living,* Spring 2012, 43.

[14] Dr. Mercola, "Child Have ADHD? Stop Feeding Them This," November 2, 2011. Viewed online at
http://articles.mercola.com/sites/articles/archive/2011/11/02/gluten-contribute-to-adhd.aspx on 12.13.12.

[15] Ibid.

[16] Ibid.

[17] Ibid.

[18] Heidi Stevenson, "The First Line of Defense Against ADHD: Eliminate Grains and Dairy," February 21, 2010. Viewed online at http://www.gaia-health.com/articles151/000181-the-first-line-of-defense-against-adhd-eliminate-grains-and-dairy.shtml on 12.13.12.

[19] Dr. Mercola, "Child Have ADHD? Stop Feeding Them This," November 2, 2011. Viewed online at
http://articles.mercola.com/sites/articles/archive/2011/11/02/gluten-contribute-to-adhd.aspx on 12.13.12.

Made in the USA
Lexington, KY
16 August 2017